POST PREGNANCY FITNESS

A guide for women over age 30, who desire to stay fit.

Sharon Roberts

Table of contents

INTRODUCTION

Welcome to "Post-Pregnancy Fitness" – the book where age and motherhood blend seamlessly with the pursuit of health and vitality.

If you're over 30 and looking to reclaim your body confidence after childbirth, you've picked the right guide.

This book isn't just about losing weight; it's about embracing a lifestyle that enhances your well-being, balances your physical fitness, and celebrates the journey of motherhood.

Here, you'll find not only workouts tailored to your unique needs, but also motivational insights and nutritional advice to support you every step of the way.

Let's embark on this transformative journey together, where every chapter brings you closer to feeling like your best self.

Bringing a new child into the world is a miraculous experience that changes a mother physically and emotionally.

Pregnancy, a wonderful yet difficult stage, ushers in an extraordinary chapter in a woman's life.

As the body goes through remarkable changes to nurture and support the developing baby, it's critical to recognize the enormous influence it has on a woman's physical and mental health.

Chapter One

What is Pregnancy?

Pregnancy, sometimes known as the miracle of life, is the miraculous process 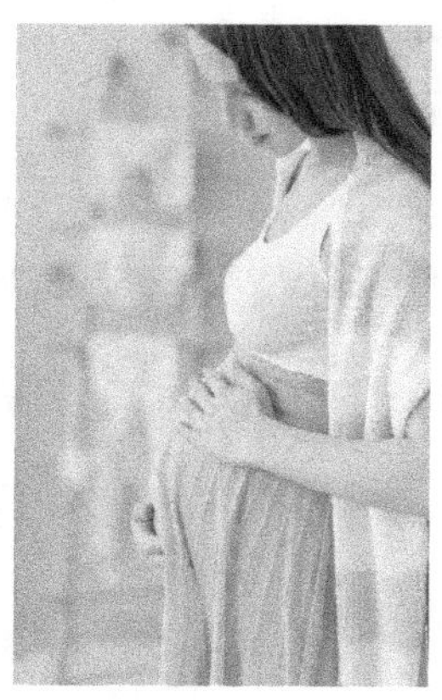 by which a fertilised egg grows into a fetus within the mother's womb. It is an era of incredible transformations, both within and outside the body. Pregnancy lasts around nine months and is filled with significant changes, hardships, and joys.

Pregnancy causes several complicated hormonal changes that help the fetus grow and thrive.

The body makes extraordinary modifications to accommodate the growing fetus, including uterine growth, hormonal changes, and changes in cardiovascular and respiratory function. Pregnancy is an emotionally charged time of expectation, excitement, and, at times, anxiety. It is a trip.

What is fitness?

Fitness is a multidimensional notion that refers to an individual's complete health and well-being, including physical, mental, and emotional components. It is not simply about being skinny or having a specific physical type, but about obtaining peak health and energy. Fitness is a mix of regular physical activity, sufficient nutrition, adequate rest, and healthy lifestyle practices.

Physical fitness is the ability to complete daily duties and activities with ease and efficiency.

It consists of several components, including cardiovascular endurance, muscular strength, flexibility, and body composition.

Regular exercise routines, such as aerobic, strength training, and flexibility exercises can improve overall physical health and quality of life.

Mental fitness is also vital, and it entails having a positive attitude, efficiently managing stress, and cultivating emotional well-being. Mindfulness meditation, relaxation practices, and seeking social support can all help improve mental fitness and resilience.

Emotional fitness refers to the ability to detect and handle emotions in a healthy and useful way. It entails developing self-awareness, coping strategies, and interpersonal interactions. Building emotional intelligence and making meaningful connections with people are critical components of emotional wellness.

Fitness has a special significance in the post-pregnancy environment, as women face the obstacles of regaining strength, energy, and confidence following childbirth.

It entails dealing with the physical changes that occur during pregnancy and childbirth, as well as the emotional transitions and duties of parenting.

After Pregnancy: A Revolutionary Experience

Post-pregnancy, sometimes referred to as the postpartum phase, is the time after childbirth when a woman's body continues to heal and adjust.

While the mother is the primary focus throughout pregnancy, the post-pregnancy phase returns attention to her as she starts the process of healing on both a physical and emotional level.

As women transition into their new roles as mothers and begin the adventure of caring for their children, the postpartum period is marked by a multitude of changes, challenges, and joys.

As the body moves from pregnancy to postpartum, it goes through a slow process of healing and rehabilitation

The uterus gradually shrinks back to its pre-pregnancy size, which is one of the most notable physical changes that women go through after giving birth.

Over several weeks, the uterus contracts and repositions itself within the pelvis, a process known as involution.

During the postpartum phase, women may also see changes in their weight, body composition, and general level of physical fitness. Some women may lose pregnancy weight fast, while others may find it difficult to reduce their weight and get back to their pre-pregnancy level of fitness.

Women have emotional ups and downs throughout the postpartum period as they adjust to the highs and lows of motherhood. Moments of weariness, self-doubt, and overwhelm are frequently punctuated by feelings of joy, love, and fulfilment.

The pressures of caring for a baby combined with the hormonal changes that happen during this time can exacerbate mood swings, anxiety, and postpartum blues.

Having self-care, patience, and support from loved ones are essential for navigating the postpartum path.

As they set out on the road to postpartum recovery and fitness, women must put their physical and mental health first.

The purpose of this guide is to give women over 30 useful tactics, advice, and tools to help them reach their post-pregnancy fitness objectives and restore their health and energy.

We will cover a wide range of post-pregnancy fitness themes in the upcoming chapters, such as suggested exercise regimens, dietary advice, self-care techniques, and methods for handling typical postpartum difficulties. This book will provide you the tools to

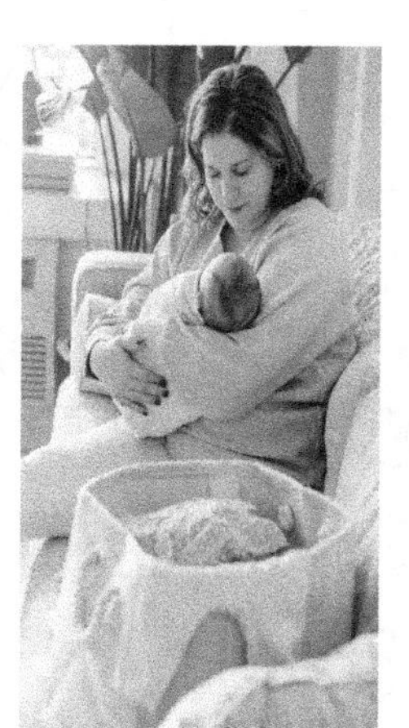

gracefully, resiliently, and confidently face your postpartum journey—whether you're a first-time mother or an experienced one.

Prepare to set out on a life-changing journey to become a happier, healthier version of yourself!

Chapter Two

Understanding Post-Pregnancy Fitness

A woman's life transforms throughout the post-pregnancy period, sometimes referred to as the postpartum period.

Her body goes through incredible changes when she becomes a mother, changes that need to be treated with kindness, care, and attention.

Women must comprehend post-pregnancy fitness when they set out to restore their health, energy, and self-assurance following childbirth.

The Postpartum Body: A Developing Structure

A woman's body goes through amazing changes throughout pregnancy to support the growth and development of the unborn child.

Pregnancy profoundly affects every element of a woman's physiology, from the uterus's growth to the weight distribution and blood volume increase. But childbirth is not the end of the changes.

The body starts the process of postpartum recovery and mending right after giving birth.

A progressive return to pre-pregnancy status characterises this phase, which is sometimes referred to as the fourth trimester.

As the body gets rid of extra fluid and tissue that is collected during pregnancy, the uterus experiences involution and eventually shrinks back to its pre-pregnancy size.

Achieving one's pre-pregnancy weight or form is only one aspect of post-pregnancy fitness, though. It's about healing the body back to health and vigour and accepting the changes that come with becoming a mother. After giving birth, women's bodies are still developing, so they must approach fitness with kindness, patience, and reasonable expectations.

Challenges in Post-Pregnancy Fitness

Regaining fitness after giving birth has its own set of difficulties. As they work to put their health and well-being first,

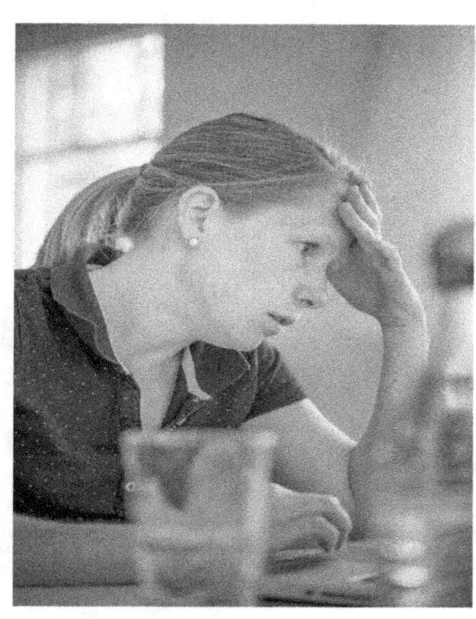

new mothers frequently encounter a variety of challenges, from physical discomfort to hormonal changes and lack of sleep.

The separation of the abdominal muscles during pregnancy, known as diastasis recti, is one of the most prevalent problems that postpartum mothers encounter. After giving delivery, this separation may continue, resulting in lower back pain, bulging belly, and core weakness.

To strengthen the core and restore abdominal integrity, diastasis recti requires specific exercises and rehabilitation methods.

Pelvic floor dysfunction, which can cause urinary incontinence, pelvic pain, and sexual discomfort, is another issue that many new mothers deal with. The pelvic floor muscles are severely strained during pregnancy and childbirth, which can result in weakening and dysfunction. Exercises for the pelvic floor, like pelvic tilts and Kegels, can help strengthen these muscles and alleviate symptoms.

Postpartum women may encounter emotional difficulties in addition to physical ones as they adjust to the rigours of parenting.

A newborn's care demands, hormonal changes, and lack of sleep can all hurt mental health and cause anxiety, sadness, and mood swings. New moms must put self-care first and ask for help from family, friends, and medical experts.

Approaching post-pregnancy fitness

Women should approach the journey to postpartum fitness with a realistic strategy and a positive perspective, even though it may seem overwhelming at first. Women should place more importance on their general health, strength, and well-being than just weight loss or desired appearance. They should resume

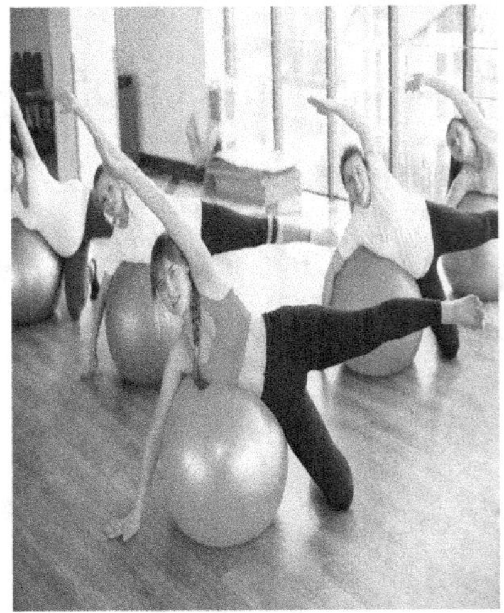

exercise after pregnancy.

1. Set Realistic Goals.

Cultivate long-term health and well-being by setting realistic and achievable goals rather than aiming for extreme body modifications or fast weight loss. Rather than obsessing over the number on the scale, concentrate on increasing strength, boosting energy, and improving general fitness.

2. Start Exercising Gradually:

After giving birth, return to exercise gradually and pay attention to your body, as your strength and endurance return, start with easy workouts like pilates, yoga, or walking, and then progressively increase the duration and intensity. Don't engage in high-impact activities or intense exercise regimens until your healthcare provider has given the all-clear.

3. Give Pelvic Floor and Core Health First Priority:

To address common postpartum concerns like diastasis recti and pelvic floor dysfunction, concentrate on strengthening the muscles of the core and pelvic floor. Include activities in your workout program that are specifically designed to target these areas, such as transverse abdominal exercises, Kegels, and pelvic tilts.

4. Embrace a Functional Fitness:

Choose functional training movements that enhance daily functioning and replicate real-life activities over isolated exercises or conventional gym sessions. Include exercises that work your entire muscle group and improve your coordination, balance, and stability.

5. Pay Attention to Your Body:

Observe how your body reacts to exercise and modify your regimen as necessary, reduce the intensity of your workouts, or make necessary modifications if you feel pain, discomfort, or exhaustion. Never forget that any exercise regimen must include relaxation and rehabilitation, particularly in the postpartum time.

6. Fuel Your Body Properly:

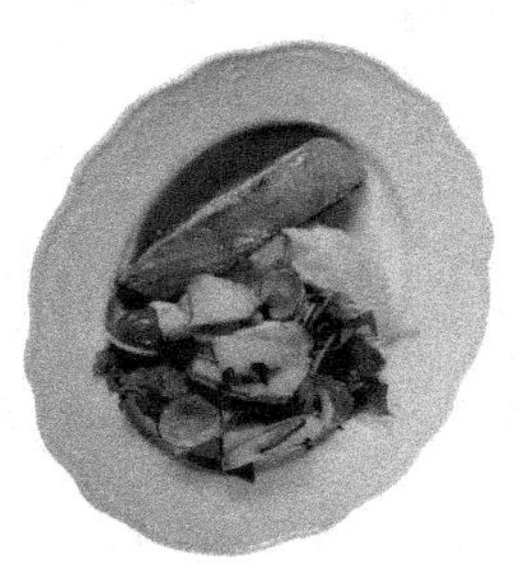

A balanced diet full of nutritious foods, lean proteins, fruits, veggies, and healthy fats will nourish your body.

Make an effort to feed your body nutrient-dense foods that promote general health, recuperation, and energy levels.

Drink plenty of water and refrain from severe calorie restrictions or diets, particularly if you are nursing.

7. Practice Self Care:

Make self-care activities that support mental health, stress relief, and relaxation a priority.

Make time for the things that make you happy and relaxed, like having a hot bath, meditating mindfully, or going for a stroll through the outdoors. Recall that to be the greatest parent you can be for your child, you must take care of yourself.

8. Look for Assistance:

As you manage the hurdles of post-pregnancy fitness, don't be afraid to ask for help from your partner, family, friends, or medical professionals. Assemble a network of people who will support you and who can provide you with advice, motivation, and hands-on help when needed.

Vicky's narrative and strengths as a 33-year-old woman

There once lived a woman by the name of Vicky in a busy metropolis full of the daily commotions of life.

Vicky was a lively and enthusiastic lady in her early thirties who had just given birth to her first child and was adjusting to the pleasures and difficulties of parenting.

Vicky was overcome with wonder at the miracle of life and the amazing trip she had on as she looked lovingly at her newborn baby. But amid the excitement and wonder of being a mother for the first time, Vicky discovered that she had to confront a problem that many women have: the desire to get back to her pre-pregnancy fitness level and shed the weight she had gained.

She set out on a path of empowerment and metamorphosis, resolved to put her health and well-being first for both herself and her expanding family. She looked for tools and advice to help her deal with the particular difficulties of maintaining her health after giving birth, and she eventually came across a thorough manual designed especially for women over thirty on how to shed pounds and regain her energy after giving birth.

The Beginning of a New Chapter

In the first section of her trip, Vicky studied the fundamentals of exercise after giving birth and discovered how crucial it was to recognize her body's requirements and limitations to restore her health and energy.

She learned that being postpartum fit meant accepting the changes that occur with being a mother and nurturing her body back to health and strength rather than just focusing on weight loss or obtaining a specific body type.

Vicky tackled her fitness path with patience, self-compassion, and a sense of empowerment after gaining this newfound insight.

She faced the difficulties of getting back into shape after giving birth, and she discovered how to prioritise self-care, set reasonable objectives, and ask for help from family and medical professionals.

Getting Through the Obstacles

Vicky faced several obstacles on her path, including mental turmoil, sleep loss, and hormonal swings in addition to physical suffering. She drew strength from the knowledge that she was not alone in her challenges and that there were tools and techniques available to help her overcome barriers, but she remained strong and determined.

She gained knowledge of the typical problems that women have after giving birth, including diastasis recti, pelvic floor dysfunction, and hormone imbalances. She also learned useful techniques and exercises to deal with these problems and encourage healing and recovery.

One step at a time, Vicky regained her strength, vitality, and confidence with persistence and determination.

Accepting the Journey

Vicky accepted the process of self-discovery and transformation as she proceeded deeper into her post-pregnancy fitness journey and realised that true fitness was about more than just physical strength—it was also about mental resilience, emotional stability, and spiritual development.

She discovered how to honour her own needs and limitations, pay attention to her body's signals, and take pleasure in the little successes along the road. Vicky developed a stronger sense of self-awareness and acceptance through mindfulness exercises, meditation, and introspection.

This helped her handle the highs and lows of parenthood with resilience and grace.

Finding Strength in the Community

Vicky found the group of women who shared her goals and experiences to be a source of inspiration, strength, and support along the way.As women from different walks of life joined together to support and empower one another on their path toward post-pregnancy fitness and well-being, she learned the value of sisterhood and solidarity.

Through social media, online forums, and in-person events, Vicky made connections with other mothers who experienced similar challenges, successes, and aspirations.

They reminded each other that they were stronger together than they were alone by pooling resources, exchanging counsel, and providing support for one another when things became tough.

Celebrating Success

Vicky thought back on how far she had come and the amazing transformation she had experienced, both physically and mentally, as she neared the end of her post-pregnancy fitness adventure.

She celebrated her newfound sense of empowerment and confidence that emanated from within and was amazed at the strength, resilience, and tenacity she had discovered within herself.

Vicky welcomed the next stage of her journey with open arms, a heart full of gratitude, and a revitalised attitude.

She knew she had the resources, support system, and know-how to keep preserving her health, energy, and well-being for years to come.

Vicky was excited and full of expectation as she looked to the future, knowing that the best was still to come.

Vicky's quest for postpartum fitness came to an end at this point, but her tale was far from finished.

She persisted in accepting the difficulties, acknowledging the accomplishments, and treasuring the happy and meaningful times that enriched her life with every day that went by. Vicky understood that achieving actual fitness involved a lifetime of personal development, evolution, and self-discovery rather than just reaching a certain point.

And one step at a time, she was happy to be experiencing it to the utmost.

Achieving postpartum fitness is a journey that calls for tolerance, tenacity, and self-compassion. It's about healing the body back to health and vigour and accepting the changes that come with becoming a mother.

You may regain your health and well-being after giving birth by establishing reasonable objectives, going cautiously at first, emphasising pelvic floor and core health, embracing functional exercise, paying attention to your body, feeding it well, taking care of yourself, and getting support.

As you start your journey toward post-pregnancy fitness, keep in mind that every woman's postpartum experience is different and that it's critical to respect your body's requirements and limitations.

You may accomplish your fitness objectives and succeed as a new mother if you are committed, persistent, and have an optimistic outlook.

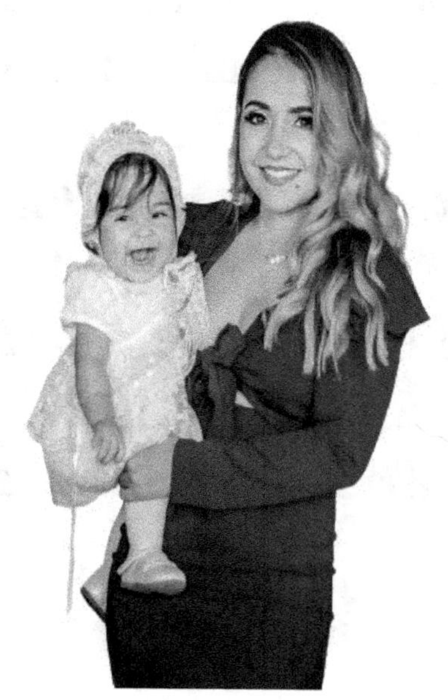

Vicky and her child living a healthy.

<u>**Motivational Insights:**</u>

Stay connected with your motivations. Whether it's wanting to play actively with your children, improving your overall health, or simply feeling good in your own skin, keep these reasons at the forefront of your mind.

When challenges arise, remind yourself why you started.

It's also helpful to set achievable goals and celebrate when you reach them, creating a positive feedback loop that keeps you motivated.

Chapter Three

Causes of Weight Gain in Women over 30 after delivering

Many women worry about gaining weight, particularly after giving birth and into their 30s.

While there is no denying that pregnancy and childbirth alter a woman's body, there are other factors that can affect weight gain during and after the postpartum period.

For ladies who want to control their weight and enhance their general health and well-being, they must comprehend these issues.

Factors Contributing to Weight Gain

Several factors can contribute to weight gain in women over 30 after delivering a baby. These include:

1. **Hormonal Changes**: A woman's body experiences notable hormonal changes during pregnancy and childbirth. The regulation of metabolism, hunger, and fat accumulation is greatly aided by

hormones like cortisol, estrogen, and progesterone.

Hormone levels may remain high or change after giving birth, which could impact energy balance and appetite control and result in weight gain.

2. Insufficient Sleep: New mothers sometimes experience sleep loss, particularly in the early postpartum period when newborns wake up a lot at

night. 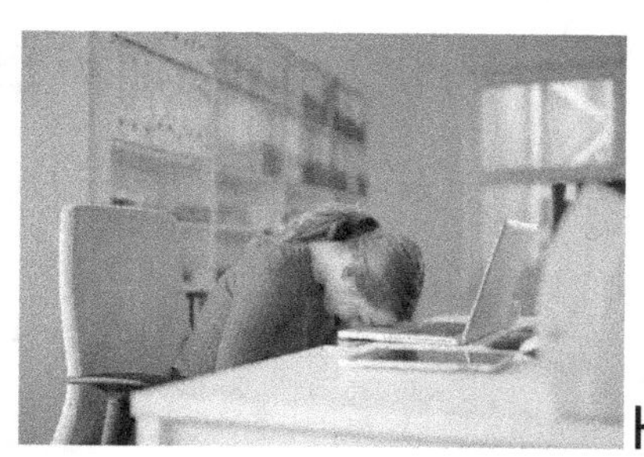 Hormonal imbalance brought on by insufficient sleep causes ghrelin, the hunger hormone, to rise and leptin, the satiety hormone, to fall, which can result in overeating and weight gain.

3. Stress: As women combine the duties of caring for a newborn, domestic obligations, employment, or other commitments, becoming a mother may be a stressful shift. Prolonged stress causes the body to release cortisol, a hormone that might encourage the storage of fat, especially in the belly area. Emotional or stress eating can also happen as a coping strategy, which can result in weight gain.

4. Lifestyle of Sedation: After giving birth, it can be difficult for women to prioritise physical activity due to the obligations of parenting, exhaustion, and time constraints. Prolonged sitting or inactivity are examples of sedentary behaviour that can lead to weight gain and metabolic disorders. In addition, if consistent physical exercise is not maintained, decreasing muscle mass and metabolic rate may happen.

5. Poor Dietary Choices: It can be difficult to strike a balance between eating a healthy diet and taking care of a newborn, so some women turn to

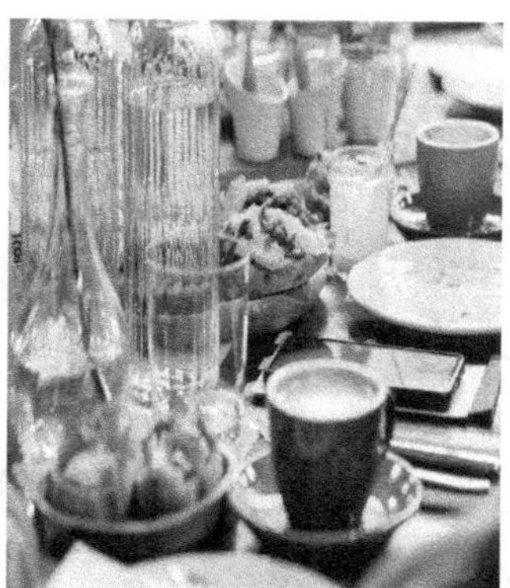

convenience foods that are heavy in calories, sugar, and bad fats.

Unhealthy eating habits, such as consuming large amounts of processed food, sugary snacks, and fast food, can lead to nutritional inadequacies and weight gain.

6. Changes in Metabolism: Changes in insulin sensitivity, glucose metabolism, and lipid metabolism are just a few of the long-lasting impacts that pregnancy and childbirth can have on a woman's metabolism. After giving birth, these metabolic alterations may last, making women more susceptible to weight gain, insulin resistance, and metabolic syndrome. This is especially true if lifestyle factors like nutrition and exercise are not sufficiently taken care of.

7. Genetic Predisposition: A woman's propensity to gain weight and become obese can also be influenced by her genetic makeup.

Regardless of lifestyle circumstances, some women may be genetically predisposed to store fat more readily or to metabolic abnormalities that cause weight gain.

Knowing one's genetic risk factors can assist guide customised weight-management strategies.

Effects of Gaining Too Much Weight

A woman's health and well-being can be seriously impacted by excessive weight gain, especially as she approaches her 30s and beyond. The following are a few consequences of excessive weight gain:

1. Increased Risk of Chronic Diseases: Gaining too much weight, particularly abdominal obesity, is linked to a higher chance of developing chronic illnesses

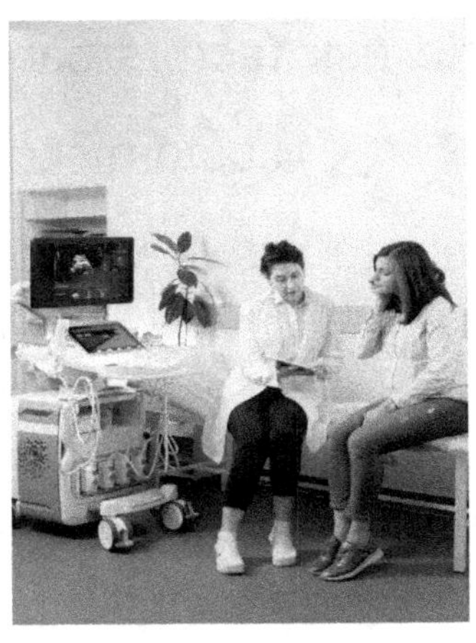

such as type 2 diabetes, heart disease, hypertension, and several cancers. Women are more susceptible to metabolic dysfunction, insulin resistance, and inflammation due to the buildup of visceral fat surrounding their organs.

2. Hormonal Imbalance: Hormones and cytokines produced by adipose tissue, or fat cells, control several bodily physiological functions. Obesity—especially fat around the abdomen—can throw off the balance of hormones, resulting in irregular menstruation cycles, infertility, and hormonal diseases including polycystic ovarian syndrome (PCOS). A vicious cycle of weight gain and metabolic dysfunction can be exacerbated by hormonal abnormalities.

3. Mental Health Problems: A woman's emotional and mental health may suffer as a result of excessive weight gain. Depression, low self-esteem, and body image issues are prevalent in women who experience weight issues. These mental health problems can be exacerbated by negative cultural attitudes toward body size and appearance, which can result in feelings of guilt, shame, and social isolation.

4. Diminished Life Quality: Being overweight can negatively affect a woman's quality of life by impairing her physical functioning, vitality, and mobility. Commonplace tasks like walking, stair climbing, and playing with kids could get harder. Obese or overweight people also frequently experience chronic discomfort, exhaustion, and sleep difficulties, which further lowers their quality of life.

5. Complications in Pregnancy: Gaining too much weight before or during a pregnancy might raise the mother's and the unborn child's risk of experiencing pregnancy difficulties. Preeclampsia, gestational diabetes, and caesarean deliveries are conditions that are more prevalent in overweight or obese women. Furthermore, a mother who gains too much weight during her pregnancy may put her unborn kid at risk for obesity and metabolic problems as an adult.

6. Shorter Life Expectancy: Reduced life expectancy and an increased risk of premature mortality are linked to obesity. Obese or overweight people are more likely to suffer from chronic illnesses and their complications, which can include heart attacks, strokes, and some types of cancer and lower life expectancy. Overall health and longevity can be enhanced by implementing healthy lifestyle practices and practising efficient weight management.

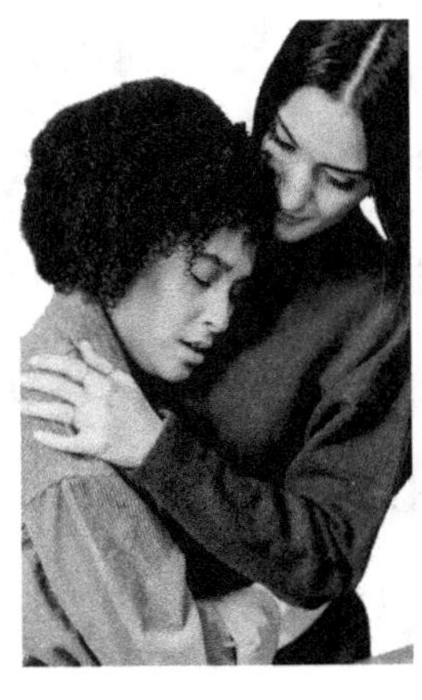

In conclusion, several factors, such as hormonal changes, sleep deprivation, stress, leading a sedentary lifestyle, making poor food choices, metabolic changes, and genetic predisposition, can all have an impact on weight gain in women over 30 who have recently given birth.

Gaining too much weight can be harmful to a woman's health and well-being because it raises her risk of mental health problems, hormone imbalances, chronic diseases, lower quality of life, difficult pregnancies, and shorter lifespans.

To maintain a healthy weight and improve their general health and well-being

Before and after childbirth, women must place a high priority on healthy lifestyle practices, including regular exercise, a balanced diet, stress reduction, and enough sleep.

Motivational Insights:

As you embark on your post-pregnancy fitness journey, remember that every small step counts towards your larger goal of well-being. It's not just about shedding pounds but about building strength—both physically and mentally. Embrace the process and celebrate your progress, no matter how incremental.

Regaining Fitness and Weight Loss after Delivering

A typical objective for many women who have recently given birth is to lose weight and regain fitness.

But the postpartum phase brings special problems of its own, mental and physical, that need careful thought and preparation.

Women can safely and sustainably reach their health and well-being objectives by putting into practice smart postpartum weight reduction techniques and efficient ways of regaining fitness. After giving birth, regaining fitness calls for a methodical, all-encompassing strategy that takes into account the special requirements of the postpartum body. The following are some methods to assist women in getting back to their pre-pregnancy levels of fitness:

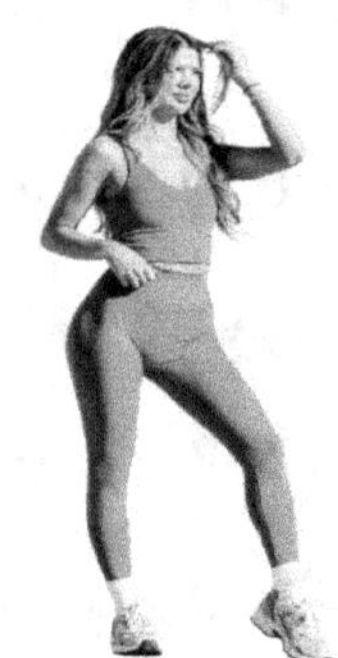

1. Start carefully: When returning to physical exercise after giving birth, it's important to pay attention to your body and go carefully. Start with easy activities like yoga, walking, or postpartum workouts that are meant to help you regain your strength and endurance. Wait to engage in strenuous exercise or high-impact activities until your healthcare provider gives the all-clear.

2. Emphasise Pelvic Floor and Core Exercises: The core and pelvic floor muscles might become weaker during pregnancy and childbirth, which can result in problems including diastasis recti and pelvic floor dysfunction.

Enhance stability, support, and function by incorporating exercises designed to target these areas into your workout program, such as transverse abdominal exercises, Kegels, and pelvic tilts.

3. Incorporate Strength Training: Increasing muscle mass is essential for increasing overall fitness, body composition, and metabolism. Include strength training activities to target main muscle groups and improve tone and strength. You can use body weight, resistance bands, or free weights. Emphasise functional motions that enhance daily functionality by imitating real-life activities.

4. Include Cardiovascular Exercise:
Walking, running, cycling, or swimming are examples of cardiovascular exercises that are vital for strengthening the heart, burning calories, and building endurance. As your fitness level rises, start with low-impact exercises and progressively increase the duration and intensity. Health standards encourage engaging in at least 150 minutes of moderate-intensity aerobic exercise every week.

5. Adopt a Functional Fitness Lifestyle:
Postpartum women can benefit greatly from functional fitness exercises, which emphasise motions that increase strength, balance, coordination, and

flexibility. Include actions that resemble everyday tasks in your workouts, such as planks, squats, lunges, and modified push-ups, to increase your general functional capacity and lower your chance of injury.

6. Maintain Hydration: For general health and fitness, adequate hydration is crucial, particularly in the postpartum phase when the body is healing from childbirth and nursing. To stay hydrated and promote the best possible physical performance, energy levels, and recuperation, drink lots of water throughout the day.

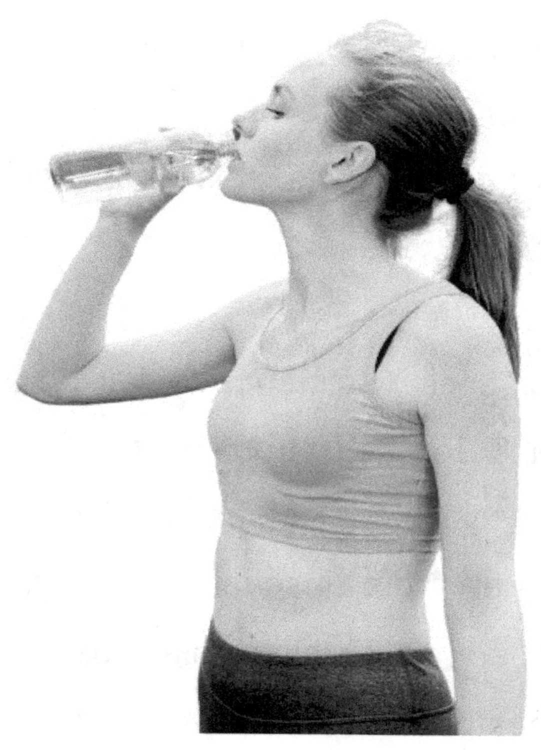

7. Make Rest and Recovery a Priority:

Sufficient rest and recuperation are crucial elements of any fitness regimen, especially in the postpartum phase when weariness and lack of sleep are prevalent. To promote recovery and avoid overtraining, pay attention to your body's cues and give restorative exercises like foam rolling, gentle stretching, and relaxation techniques priority.

8. Seek Assistance: Never be afraid to ask for help from a certified fitness specialist or personal trainer, who can offer you inspiration, support, and customised training plans based on your postpartum requirements and objectives. Joining an online group or postpartum fitness class can offer accountability, support, and companionship on your fitness journey.

Regaining fitness after pregnancy is a gradual process, and it's essential to focus on a balanced approach that supports both physical recovery and adequate nutrition. Here are some key nutritional guidelines to consider:

1. **Calorie Intake:** After pregnancy, your calorie needs might slightly decrease compared to during pregnancy, but if you're breastfeeding, you'll still need about 300-500 extra calories per day. It's important that these calories come from nutrient-rich foods to help your body recover and provide quality breastmilk.

2. **Balanced Diet**: Aim for a diet that includes a variety of foods:

- Proteins: Lean meats, fish, eggs, dairy, beans, and legumes help repair tissue and support muscle recovery.

- Whole Grains:: Brown rice, whole wheat bread, oatmeal, and quinoa are great for energy.

- Healthy Fats:: Avocados, nuts, seeds, and olive oil can aid in healing and inflammation reduction.

- Fruits and Vegetables: A wide range ensures you get adequate vitamins, minerals, and antioxidants.

3. Moderation in Processed Foods:: Limit intake of high-sugar and high-fat processed foods, which can impede recovery and contribute to weight retention or gain.

4. **Calcium and Iron**: These are particularly important. Calcium (found in dairy products, green leafy vegetables, and fortified foods) is vital for bone health, while iron (found in lean meats, beans, and fortified cereals) is crucial for energy and preventing anaemia.

5. **Vitamins such as D and B12**: These are important for your own health and for breastfeeding.

Vitamin D can be sourced from sunlight and fortified foods or supplements; B12 is found in animal products or supplements, especially important for vegetarians and vegans.

6. **Avoid Alcohol and Limit Caffeine**::
Alcohol can interfere with breastfeeding and recovery, and excessive caffeine can affect your sleep and potentially your baby's if you are breastfeeding.

Start slowly, possibly with walking or gentle postpartum exercises, and progressively increase intensity based on how you feel.

Always listen to your body and seek advice from healthcare professionals regarding diet and exercise post-pregnancy.

Tips for Losing Weight After Delivery

Many women want to reduce weight after giving birth to get back to their pre-pregnancy weight or to obtain a healthier body composition, in adondition to restoring their physical fitness. The following weight-loss advice is especially designed with the postpartum period in mind:

1. Give Nutrient-Dense Foods Special Attention:

Make a point of consuming a diet high in fruits, vegetables, lean meats, whole grains, and healthy fats to provide your body with the resources it needs to support weight loss and general wellness. Steer clear of overly processed foods, sugary snacks, and empty calories as these may exacerbate nutrient shortages and weight gain.

2. Practice Portion Control: To prevent overeating and encourage weight loss, pay attention to portion sizes and engage in mindful eating. To avoid consuming extra calories, use smaller plates, gauge serving sizes, and pay attention to your body's signals of hunger and fullness.

3. Eat Regularly: To maintain energy levels, reduce cravings, and stabilise blood sugar levels, aim for frequent, well-balanced meals and snacks throughout the day. Going too long without eating or skipping meals might cause overindulgence and bad eating decisions later in the day.

4. Incorporate Protein into Every Meal: An important part of a postpartum weight loss diet, protein is necessary for muscle regeneration, satiety, and metabolic function. For maximum support for muscle growth and repair, incorporate lean protein sources like fish, poultry, tofu, beans, lentils, and Greek yoghourt into each meal.

5. Stay Active: Include regular exercise in your daily routine to aid in weight loss, enhance general health, and increase fitness. To increase fat burning and support fat reduction while maintaining lean muscle mass, combine aerobic, strength, and flexibility activities.

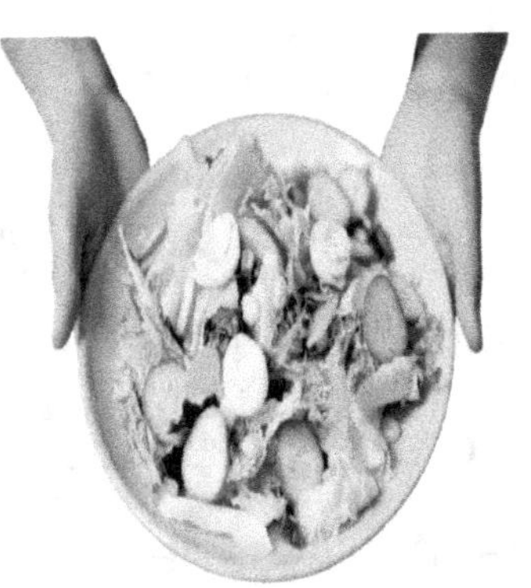

6. Engage in Mindful Eating: To create a better relationship with food, pay attention to your eating patterns and feelings. Engage in mindful eating. To avoid thoughtless and emotional eating, take your time, enjoy every bite, and pay attention to your body's signals of hunger and fullness.

7. Stay Hydrated: To help with weight reduction and to stay hydrated, drink lots of water throughout the day. Water is a

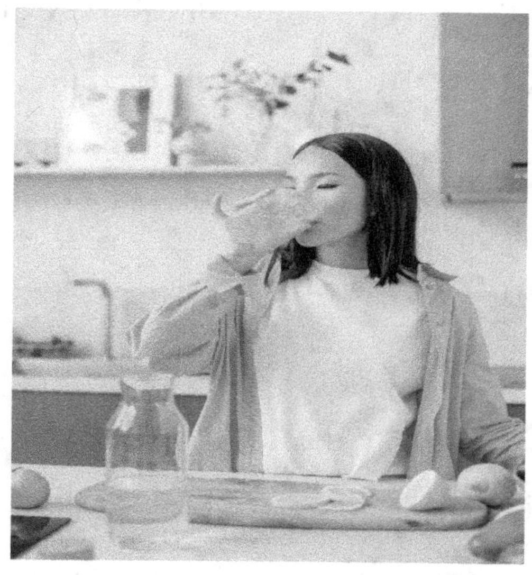

crucial part of any postpartum weight loss regimen since it can increase feelings of fullness, increase metabolism, and inhibit hunger.

8. Get Enough Sleep: To assist weight loss and general health, make sleep a priority and make sure you get enough restorative sleep every night.

Try to get between seven and nine hours of good sleep every night if you can because getting too little sleep can mess with hormone levels, increase hunger, and make it harder to lose weight.

9. Exercise Realistic Patience: Keep in mind that losing weight takes time, particularly during childbirth when the body is going through a lot of changes. Have patience with yourself and make reasonable, attainable goals that put your health and well-being before quick outcomes.

Acknowledge minor triumphs during the journey and concentrate on advancement instead of flawlessness.

In conclusion, postpartum fitness recovery and weight loss necessitate a thorough strategy that takes nutrition and activity into account.
Women can regain their strength, stamina, and confidence after giving birth by using strategies for regaining fitness, such as starting slowly, concentrating on core and pelvic floor exercises, incorporating strength training and cardiovascular exercise, embracing functional fitness, staying hydrated, prioritising rest and recovery, and seeking support.

Women can also achieve their weight loss goals and improve their overall health and well-being in the postpartum period by adhering to weight loss tips specific to the postpartum experience, such as emphasising nutrient-dense foods, exercising portion control, eating regularly, and including protein in every meal, staying active, engaging in mindful eating, drinking plenty of water, getting enough sleep, and being realistic and patient.

Women may thrive while they enjoy the joys and trials of parenting, regain their fitness, and reduce weight with commitment, consistency, and a positive outlook.

Nutritional Advice:

Fueling your body with the right nutrients is crucial, especially during this transformative period. Focus on balanced meals that include a variety of proteins, healthy fats, and carbohydrates. Hydration is key—water aids in metabolism and helps keep you feeling full, which can be beneficial for weight management.

Chapter Four

The Benefits of Regaining Fitness After Delivery

It takes more than simply reaching a specific body type or fitting into 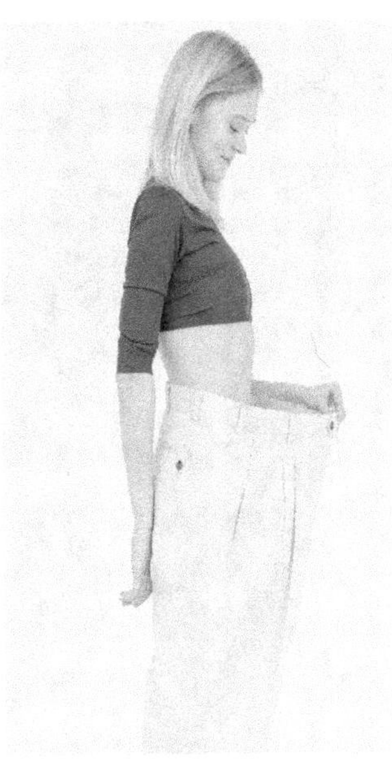 pre-pregnancy clothes to get back in shape after giving birth. Regaining your health, energy, and self-assurance while navigating the benefits and drawbacks of motherhood is the goal.

The advantages of postpartum exercise are manifold and extensive, ranging from enhancing physical strength and endurance to elevating mental health and improving general quality of life. Let's examine the advantages it provides for both physical and mental health, as well as the significance of postpartum exercise.

Importance of Post-Pregnancy Fitness

A woman's life transforms both physically and emotionally throughout the postpartum period. While caring for the growing child is frequently the main emphasis throughout pregnancy, the post-pregnancy phase returns attention to the mother as she works through the difficulties of healing, recuperation, and adjusting to parenting.

After giving birth, getting back in shape is crucial for several reasons:

1.Promote Physical Recovery: A woman's body is significantly strained during pregnancy and childbirth, which can result in abnormalities like weakening muscles, unstable joints, and problems with the pelvic floor.

Exercises for postpartum fitness increase overall mobility and function, strengthen muscles and improve flexibility, all of which aid in the physical recovery process.

2. Encourages Mental Health: Women may experience emotional difficulties during the postpartum period as they adjust to changing hormones, lack of sleep, and the responsibilities of taking care of a newborn. Exercise has been demonstrated to have strong impacts on mood, lowering levels of stress chemicals like cortisol and producing endorphins.

Regular physical activity can boost mood, reduce symptoms of anxiety and postpartum depression, and improve mental health in general.

3. Elevates Vitality: Being a parent demands an endless supply of energy, and getting back in shape after giving birth can help increase energy levels and fight off feelings of weariness and exhaustion. Exercise improves cardiovascular health and cellular energy generation by increasing blood flow and oxygen supply to tissues. Postpartum women who place a high priority on their fitness frequently express feeling more capable, awake, and enthusiastic about meeting the demands of daily living.

4. Enhances Self-Confidence: A woman's self-esteem and body image can be negatively impacted by pregnancy and childbirth, which can result in feelings of insecurity and unhappiness with one's looks.

After giving birth, getting back in shape can boost one's self-esteem and body positivity by strengthening muscles, increasing physical stamina, and encouraging a feeling of empowerment and achievement.

Women who choose a healthy, active lifestyle can feel more confident in their physical appearance and recognize their full range of potential.

5. Strengthens Bond with baby: Including exercise in regular routines will help you spend quality time with your infant and build a sense of intimacy and connection.

Whether it's taking postnatal fitness courses, doing mother and me yoga, or taking walks with your infant in the stroller together, engaging in physical activity as a family can strengthen the parent-child bond and create lasting memories.

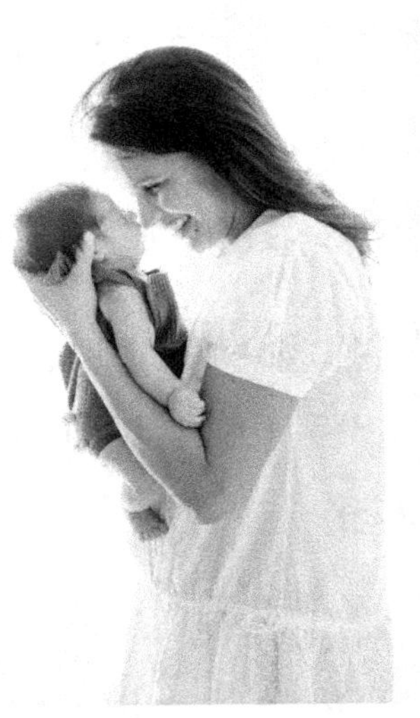

Physical Health Benefits of Post-Pregnancy Fitness

Recovery from childbirth brings several physical health advantages, as well as boosting confidence and mental well-being. The following are some ways that physical health might be enhanced by post-pregnancy fitness:

1. Strengthen Muscles and Joints:

Muscle imbalances, pelvic instability, and back discomfort are among the problems that might arise during pregnancy and childbirth, which can weaken muscles and joints. Exercises for strength training increase joint stability, strengthen muscles and lower the chance of injury. By focusing on important muscular regions including the upper body, glutes, and core, one can increase overall strength and function and facilitate and ease daily activities.

2. Enhances Cardiovascular Well-Being:

Increased blood volume, heart rate, and blood pressure are just a few of the changes that pregnancy and childbirth can cause to your cardiovascular health. Aerobic activity, like jogging, cycling, swimming, or walking, lowers blood pressure, increases cardiovascular fitness, and lowers the risk of heart disease. Frequent aerobic exercise also strengthens the heart generally, increases circulation and aids in weight loss.

3. Assists in Weight Control: Gaining weight during pregnancy is common because the body stores fat to support the developing fetus. Women who regain fitness after giving birth can better control their weight and have a balanced body composition. Exercise enhances metabolism, raises calorie expenditure, and encourages fat reduction while maintaining lean muscle mass. In addition, a healthy diet and frequent exercise are key to achieving and maintaining a healthy weight after childbirth.

4. Improves Posture and Alignment: As the body adjusts to fit the developing baby, pregnancy can cause changes to posture and alignment.

Problems including pelvic instability, muscular imbalances, and back discomfort can all be attributed to poor posture and alignment. Exercises that focus on postural awareness, spinal alignment, and core strength can help with pain management, posture correction, and overall spinal health.

5. Encourages Healthy Pelvic Floor: The pelvic floor muscles can become weaker during pregnancy and childbirth, which can result in problems like pelvic organ prolapse, incontinence, and sexual dysfunction. Exercises for the pelvic floor, like pelvic tilts and Kegels, assist in strengthening the muscles supporting the bladder and improve sexual performance. Including pelvic floor exercises in your workout regimen can help maintain the condition of your pelvic floor and prevent or relieve common postpartum issues.

Mental Health Benefits of Post-Pregnancy Fitness

Postpartum activity has several advantages for mental health in addition to its physical health benefits. Following childbirth, regular exercise can promote mental health in the following ways:

1. Reduces Tension and Fear: As women deal with the demands of caring for a child and adjusting to changes in their bodies and routines, the postpartum period can be a taxing and anxious time. 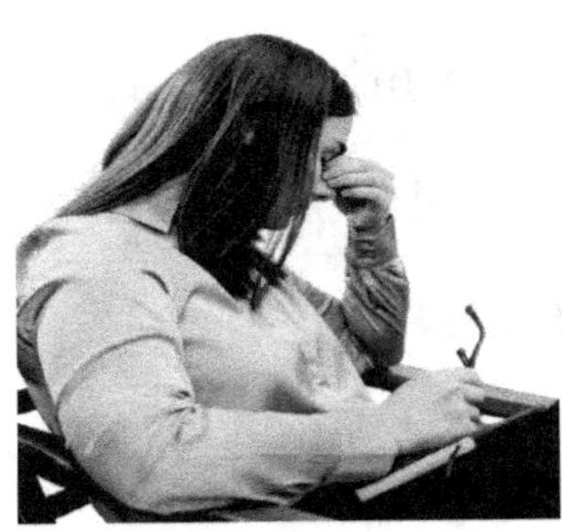 Exercise has been demonstrated to raise levels of feel-good neurotransmitters like endorphins and lower levels of stress chemicals like cortisol, which boost mood and lessen anxiety.

2. Elevates Sensation and Joy: Hormone changes brought on by pregnancy and childbirth can cause mood swings, irritability, and depressive or melancholy thoughts. Regular exercise causes the neurotransmitters dopamine, serotonin, and endorphins to be released, which in turn enhances emotions of pleasure, enjoyment, and well-being.

Exercise can enhance mood and perspective on life while reducing the symptoms of postpartum depression.

3. Boosts Confidence and Self-Esteem: Having a kid or going through a pregnancy can affect one's self-esteem and body image, which can cause feelings of insecurity and dissatisfaction with one's appearance.

Regular exercise fosters a sense of empowerment, accomplishment, and pride in one's physical capabilities, all of which can enhance one's body image and self-esteem.

Women who exercise to restore strength, endurance, and confidence frequently report improvements in their sense of overall worth and self-worth.

4. Makes Time for Personal Well-Being:

It might be difficult to find time for personal activities and self-care when raising a newborn.

Regular exercise gives women a designated time slot to focus on their own physical and mental well-being, apart from the responsibilities of parenting.

Whether you're running, heading to a fitness class, or practising yoga, exercise can serve as a form of self-care and stress relief, allowing women to recharge and rejuvenate.

5. Improves Cognitive Function: Research has indicated that exercise

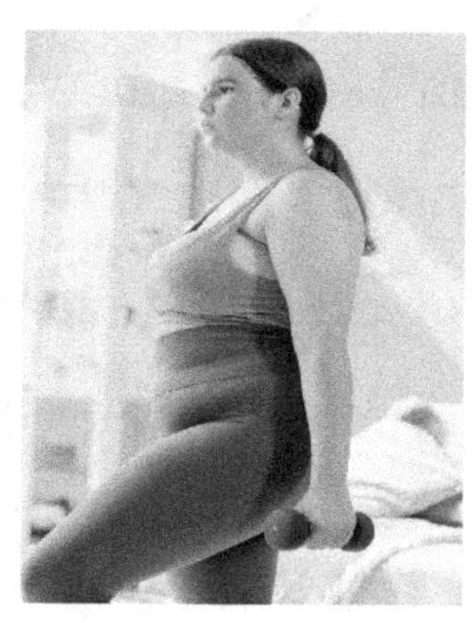

improves memory, focus, and cognitive function—all of which are advantageous for new mothers acclimating to the rigours of parenthood. Frequent exercise raises blood, boost our immune system and helps us stay healthy. Exercise can have numerous benefits for new moms. It can help with postpartum recovery, improve mood, increase energy levels, and promote better sleep. Additionally, exercise can aid in weight loss, strengthen muscles that may have weakened during pregnancy, and provide a much-needed break from the demands of caring for a newborn. Plus, engaging in physical activity can be a great way for new moms to connect with others and establish a sense of routine and self-care amidst the challenges of motherhood.

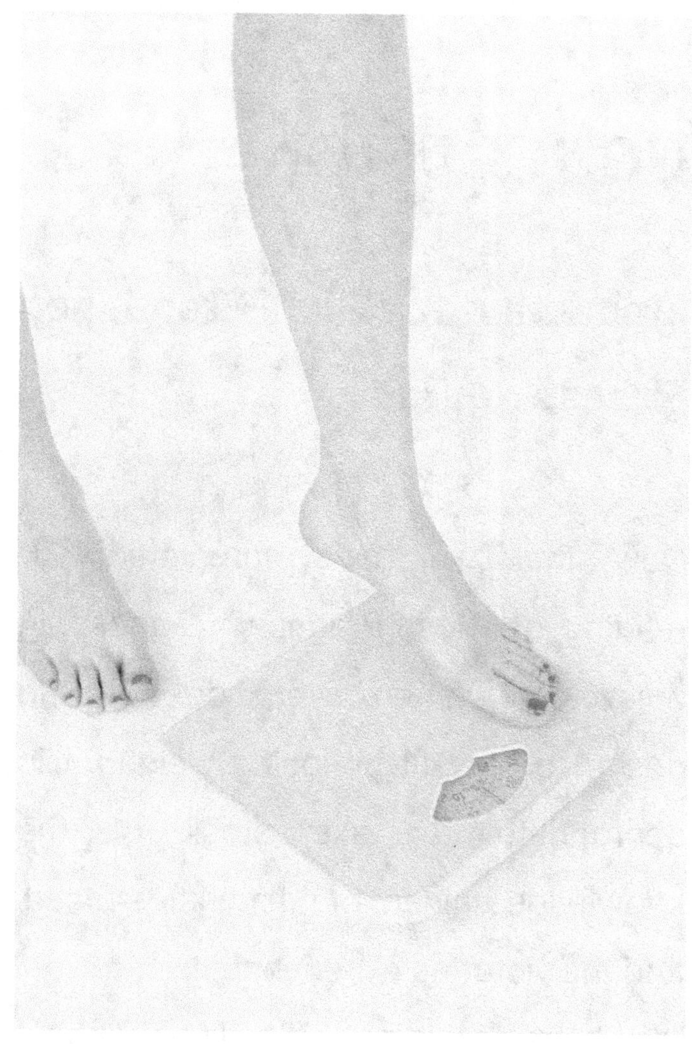

Always check your weight.

CONCLUSION

Embracing the Post-Pregnancy Fitness Journey

Now that we have completed our reading of "Post Pregnancy Fitness: A guide for women over age 30, who desire to stay fit by losing weight; it is appropriate to take stock of the knowledge gained, the difficulties faced, and the victories experienced.

We have examined the life-changing potential of postpartum fitness and its significant influence on women's experiences navigating the pleasures and difficulties of parenting throughout this extensive handbook.

We discussed the significance of comprehending the postpartum body and accepting the path of getting healthy again after giving birth in the first few chapters of our book. We discovered that regaining health, vitality, and confidence following the amazing experience of pregnancy and childbirth is the true meaning of post-pregnancy fitness, rather than merely focusing on weight loss or reaching a specific body type.

We learned about the range of difficulties that face women who have given birth, including hormonal changes, physical discomfort, lack of sleep, and emotional turmoil, as we turned through the pages of our handbook.

In addition to learning about typical problems like diastasis recti, pelvic floor dysfunction, and hormone imbalances, we also learned useful techniques and exercises to deal with these difficulties and advance healing and recovery.

We emphasised during our study the significance of establishing reasonable objectives, giving self-care priority, and asking for help from close friends and family members as well as medical experts.

We discovered that we are not alone in our problems and that there are tools and techniques available to help us get beyond obstacles, so we learned to approach post-pregnancy fitness with patience, self-compassion, and a sense of empowerment.

We welcomed the process of self-discovery and transformation as we ventured deeper into the core of postpartum fitness, realising that true fitness is about more than just physical strength—it's also about mental resilience, emotional stability, and spiritual development.

We discovered how to honour our own needs and limitations, pay attention to our bodies, and take pleasure in the little successes along the journey.

Along the journey, the group of women who shared our goals and experiences gave us bravery, strength, and support.

As women from different walks of life joined together to support and empower one another on our road toward post-pregnancy fitness and well-being,

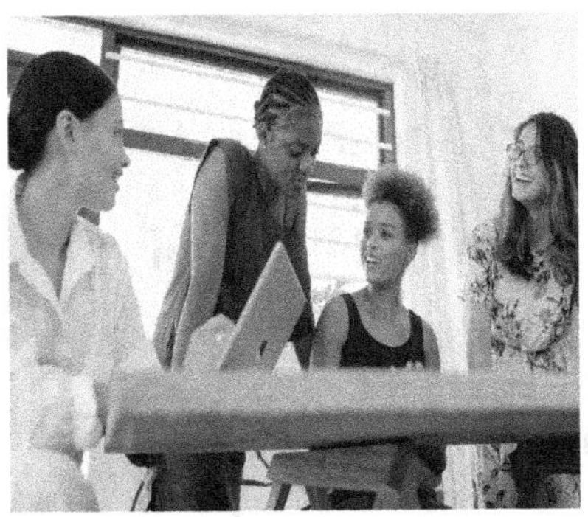

we learned the value of sisterhood and solidarity.

Let's pause as our guide comes to an end to acknowledge and appreciate the amazing physical and emotional changes we have experienced.

Let's celebrate our newfound sense of empowerment and confidence that comes from within and wonder at the strength, resilience, and determination we have found within ourselves.

However, our adventure is not over yet. Let's welcome the new chapter of our lives as we look to the future.

Embrace the trip with open arms, certain that we have the resources—including information, skills, and assistance—to maintain our health, energy, and well-being for years to come.

Let's keep embracing the difficulties, acknowledging the victories, and treasuring the happy and meaningful times that abound in our lives.

Genuine fitness is a lifetime process of development, change, and self-discovery rather than merely a goal to be attained. As we get to the end of our guidebook, let us keep in mind that as long as we continue to approach the journey with open minds and hearts, it will never really end.

Thus, cheers to the voyage that lies ahead and to you, my reader.

May it be brimming with fortitude, resiliency, and endless opportunities.

May you prosper and grow even more as you work toward becoming fit after giving birth and in the future.